For Hans.
Who stroked my bald head and giggled.

And for Anders.
Who shaved my head and told me I was beautiful.

Thousand Words Press
38 Miller Avenue, PMB #119
Mill Valley, CA 94941
415.388.2757
www.nowherehair.com

First printing 2010
First printing in paperback: 2013

Text set in Canterbury Old Style
Illustrations are watercolor
Printed in Hong Kong

ISBN-13 978-0-984-3591-3-4
ISBN-10 0-9843591-3-3
Library of Congress Control Number: 2009942025

Publisher's Cataloging-in-Publication Data

Glader, Sue Greim.
    Nowhere hair / by Sue Glader ; illustrated by Edith Buenen.
        p. cm.
    Summary : Having hunted for her mother's missing hair, a young girl learns the truth about cancer while experiencing life (with hats, scarves, baldness and love) during chemotherapy.
    ISBN 9780984359103
[1. Cancer –Fiction. 2. Chemotherapy –Fiction. 3. Medical care –Fiction. 4. Family life –Fiction. 5. Mother and child –Fiction.] I. Buenen, Edith. II. Title.

PZ7.G472 No 2010
[E]—dc22   2009942025

Manufactured through InterPress Ltd in Hong Kong
February 2013 - Job#J131037

Nowhere Hair

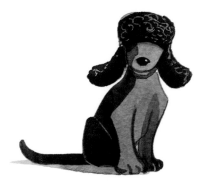

by Sue Glader
Illustrated by Edith Buenen

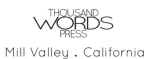
THOUSAND
WORDS
PRESS

Mill Valley . California

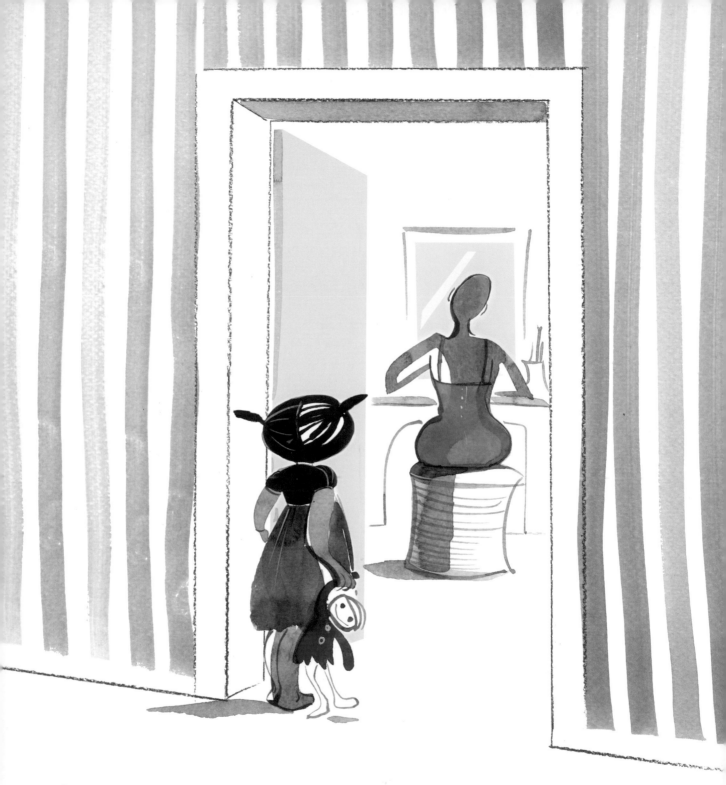

I want to know where Mommy has lost all of her hair.

Where did it go?

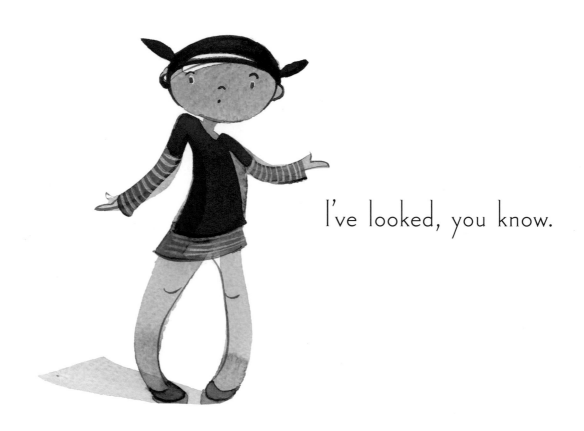

I've looked, you know.

And it's not anywhere.

She didn't hide
it in her purse.

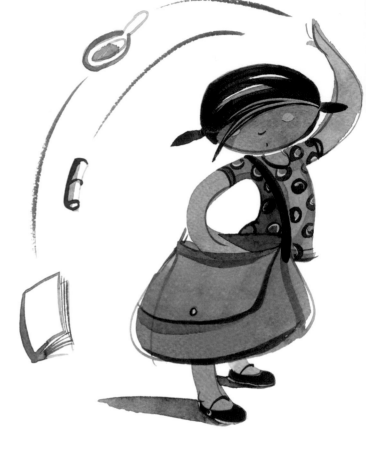

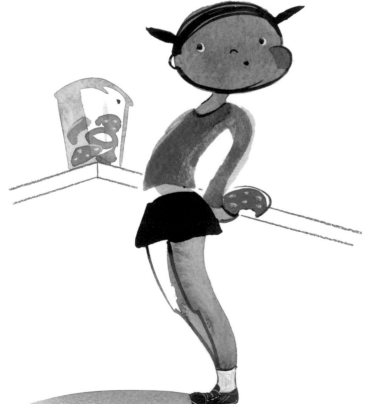

Or in the cookie jar.

I've even peeked beneath her bed.

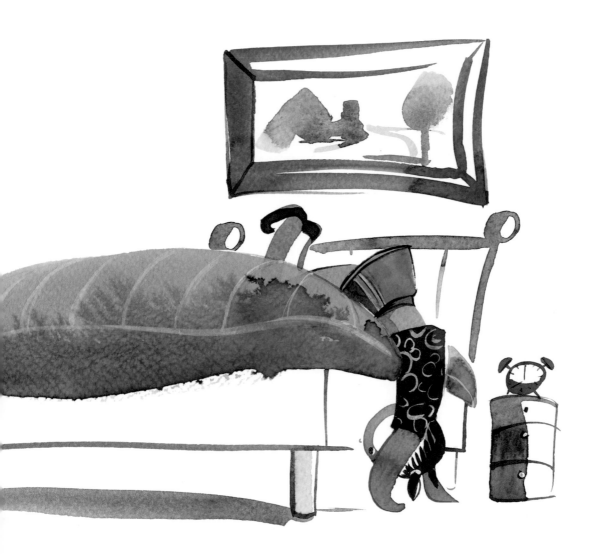

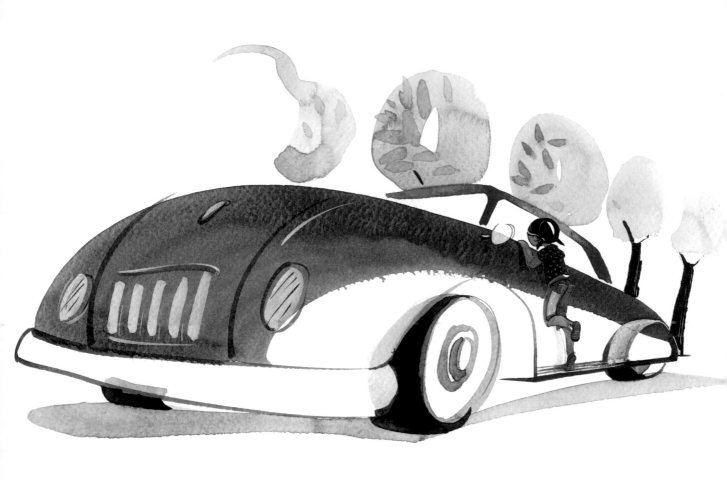

And searched our big blue car.

She could have lent it to a cat
who needed a warm cloak.

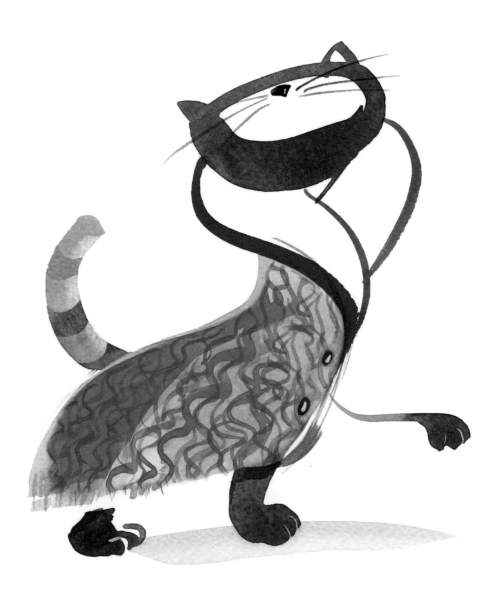

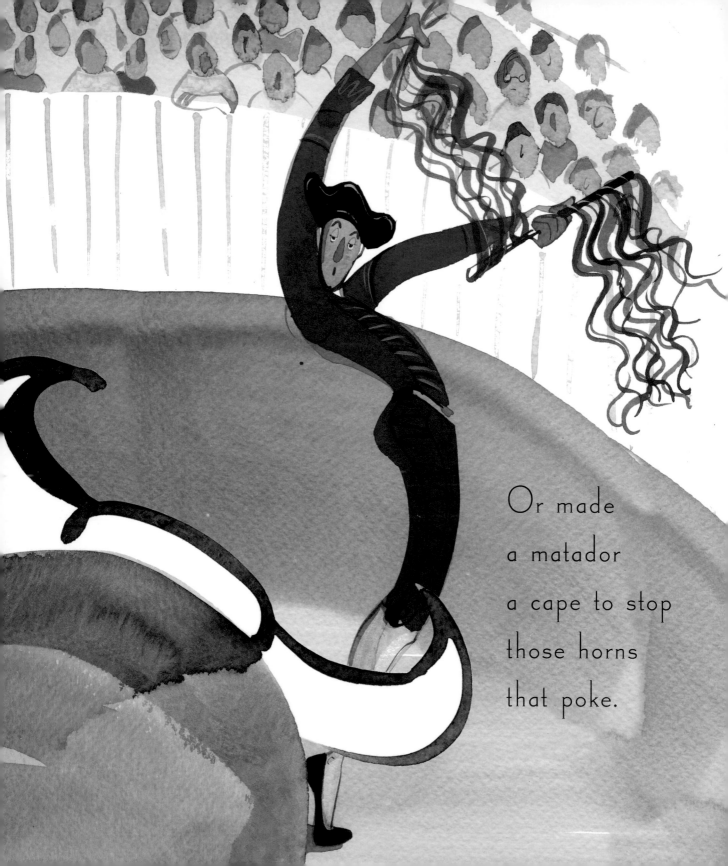

Or made
a matador
a cape to stop
those horns
that poke.

A sparrow might have borrowed it
to warm her fancy nest.

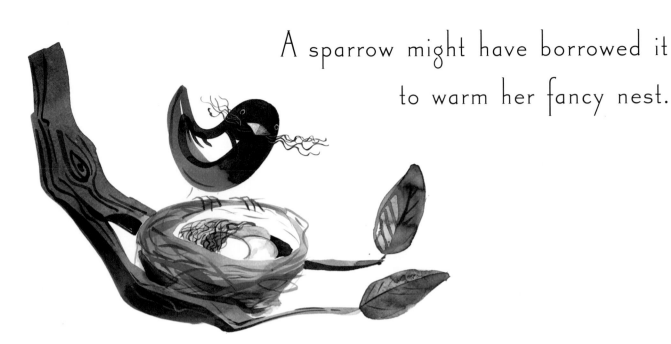

Perhaps she stuffed a pillow
to help Grandma get some rest.

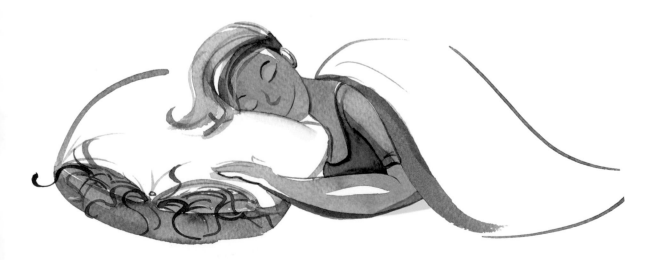

The day I asked her where it went
she had a simple answer.
"I'm bald because of medicine
I take to treat my cancer."

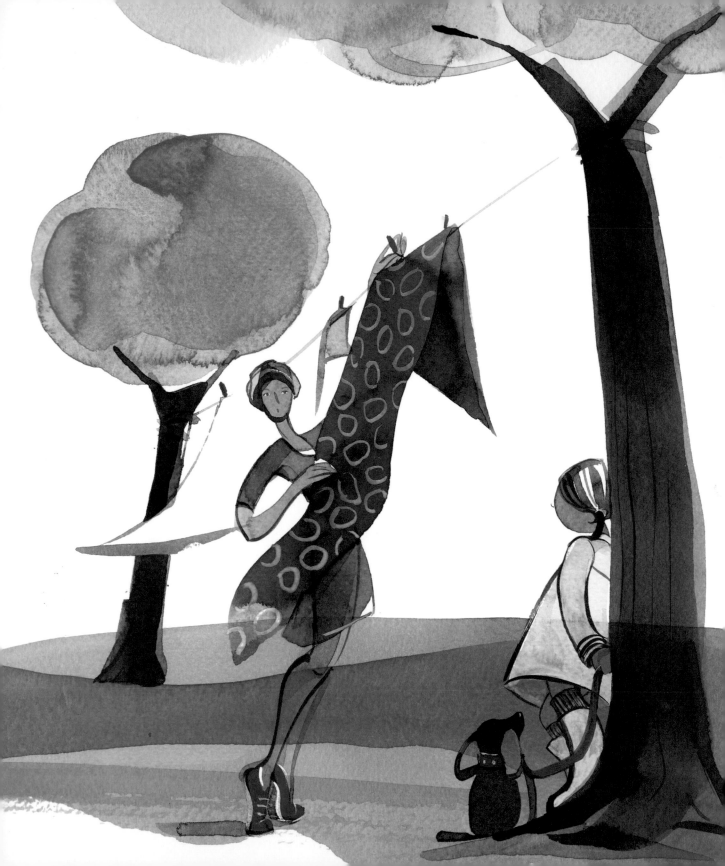

It wasn't something that I did.

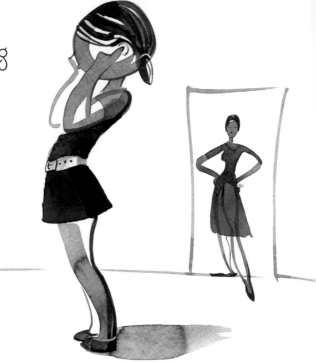

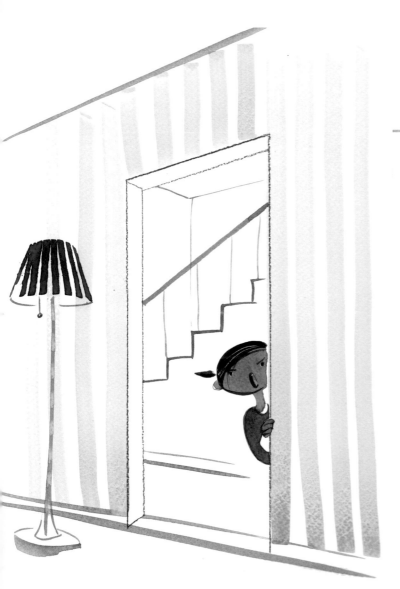

Or said.

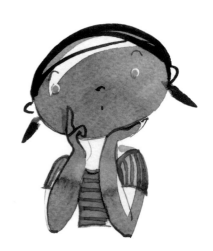

Or even thought.

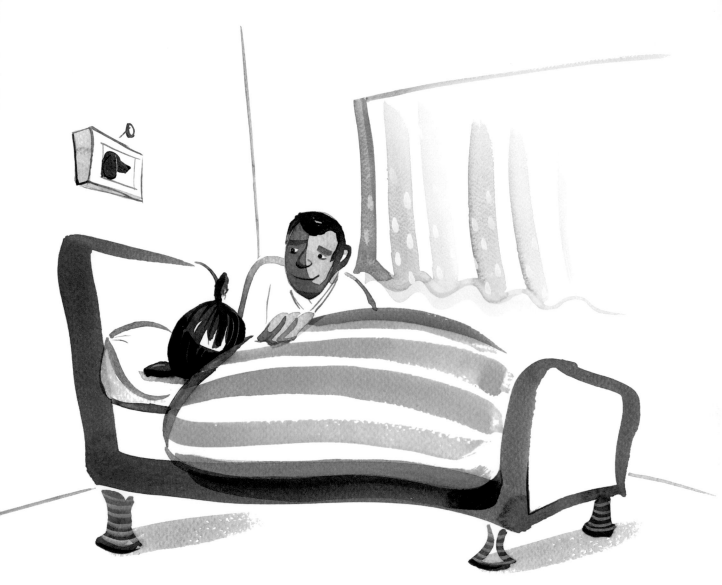

Dad promised me
(in bed last night)
it's not because we fought.

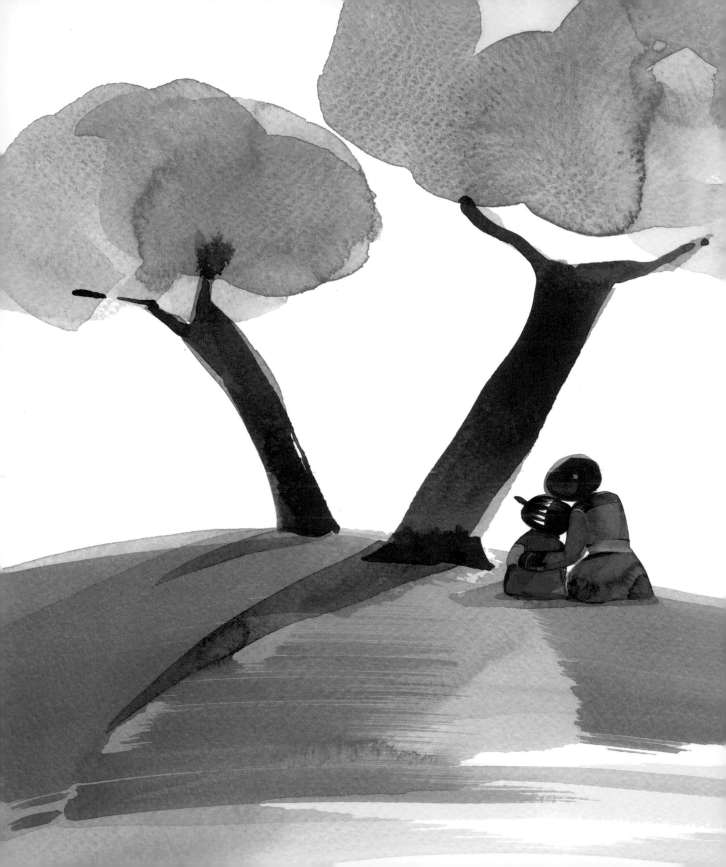

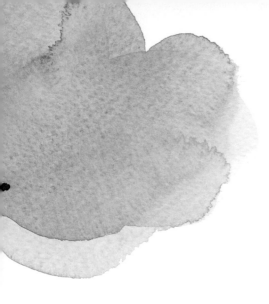

We don't get to the park as much.
Mom likes the couch a lot.
Still even when she kisses me,
I can't catch what she's got.

Having cancer
hasn't changed
the way she is
with me.

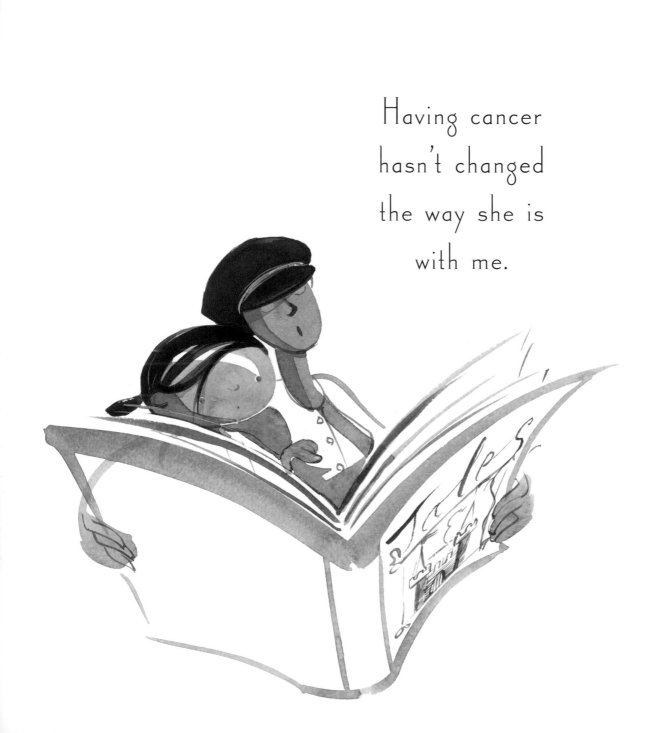

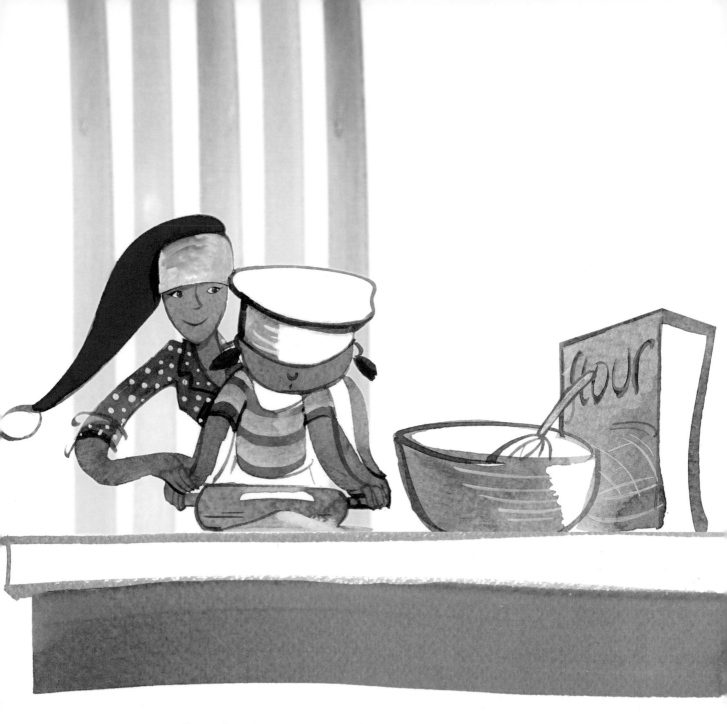

She's given me her very own
"Mom Loves You" guarantee.

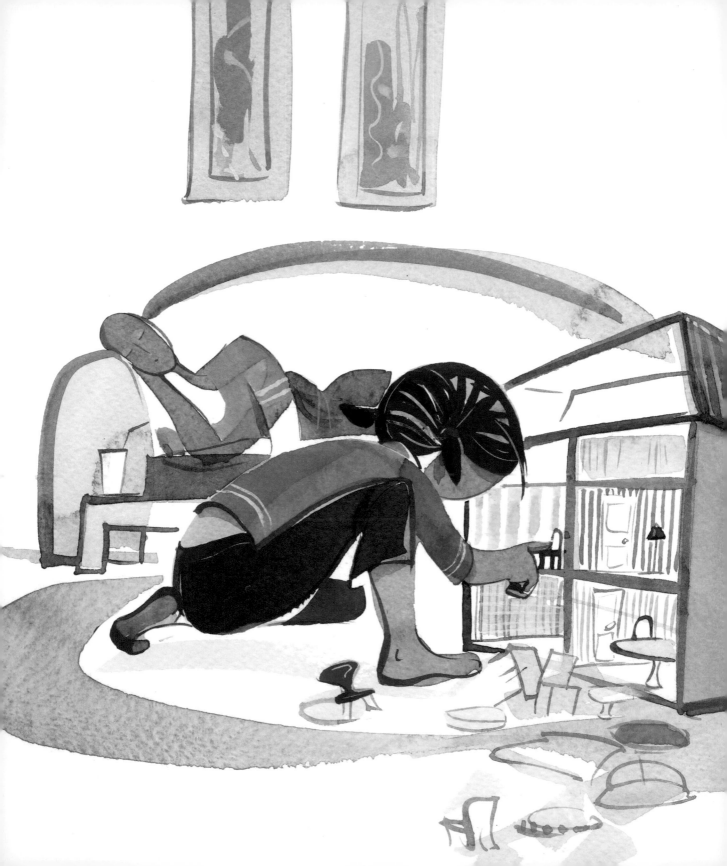

It makes me scared that she is sick.

I want her well right now.

She says, "Be patient, Little One."

That seems so hard somehow.

What's different now is all these hats.
There's one for every mood.

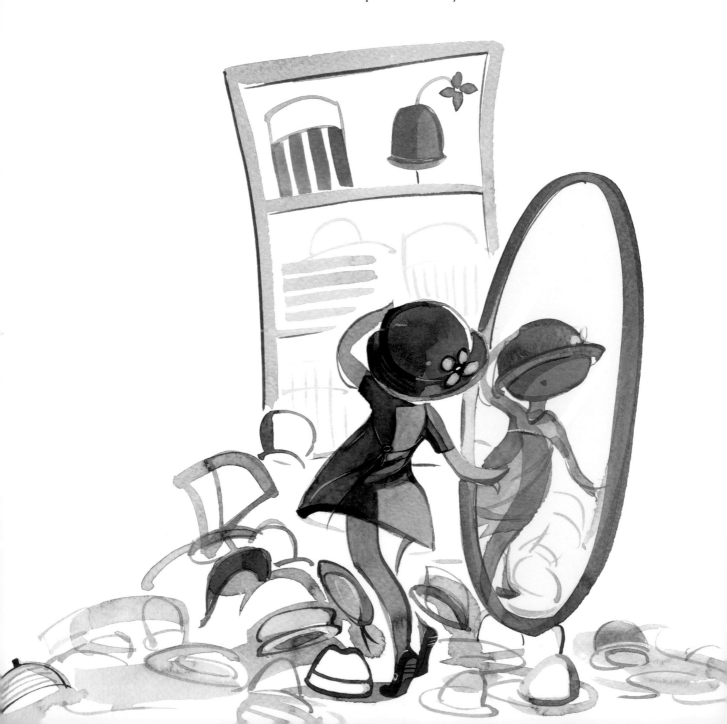

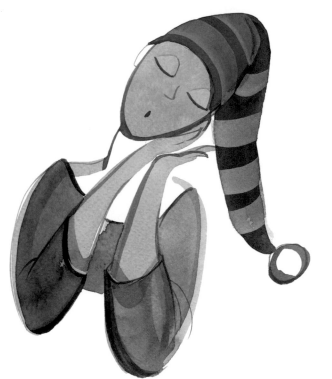

Sleepy.

Crabby.

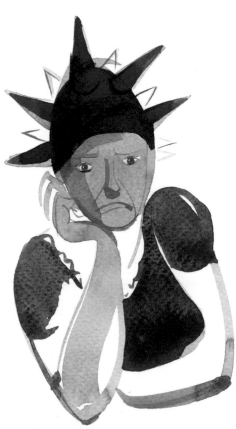

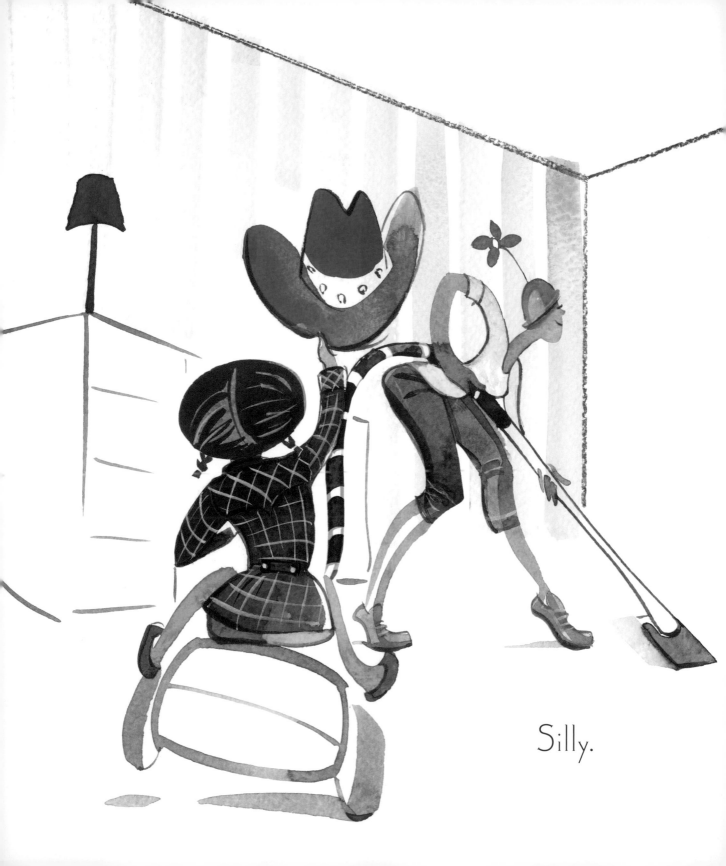

Silly.

Happy.

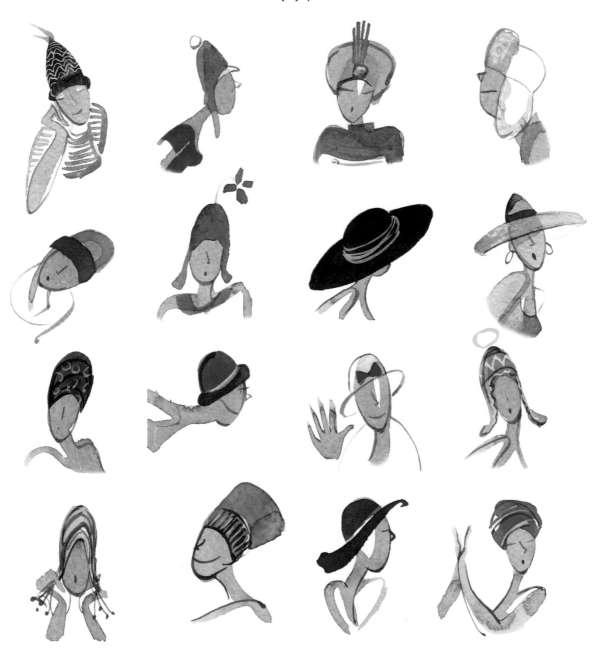

They help her attitude.

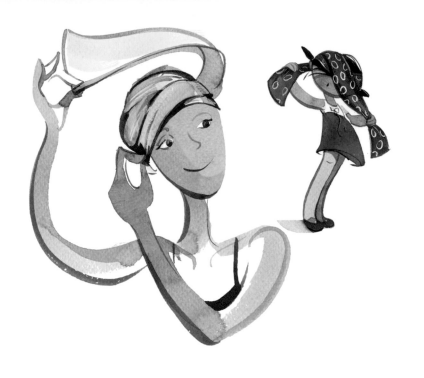

Some days
she wears
a plain turban
swirled around
her head.

I wish she bought a fancy one
with polka dots instead.

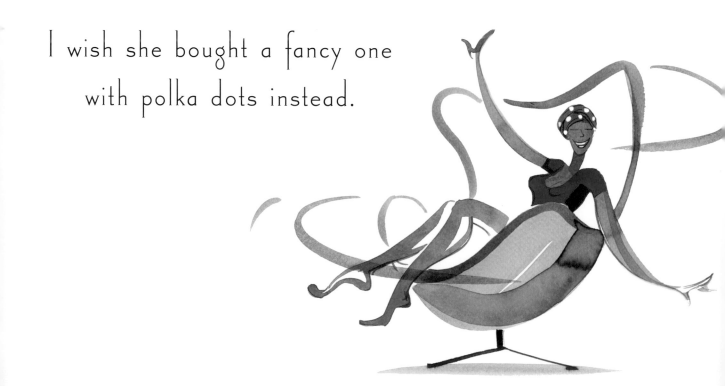

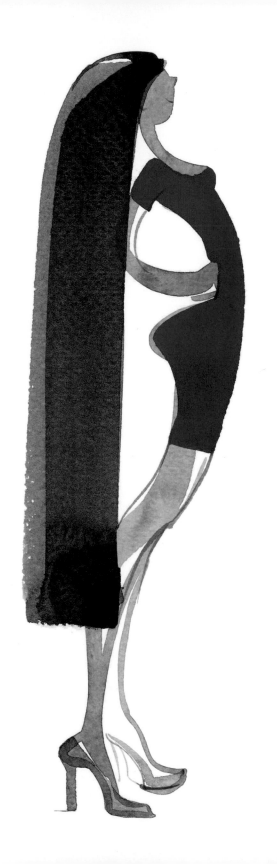

She has
a crazy wig
as well,
with
fake hair
straight
and
long.
It makes
her look
like
someone
else.
To me,
that seems
all wrong.

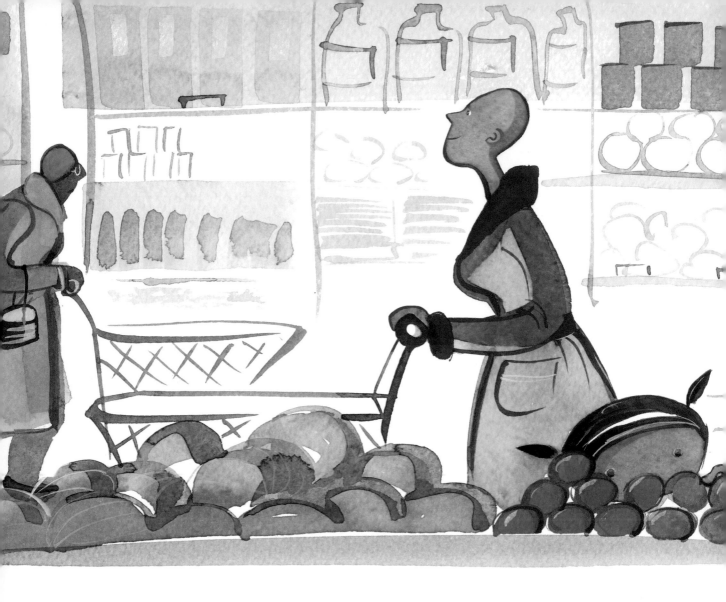

When Mommy's feeling confident,
she wears nothing at all.

She says it's like my first hairdo
when I was very small.

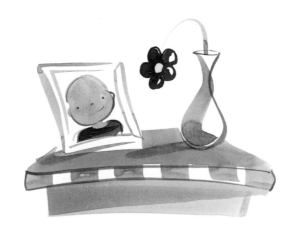

So if you see her, please be kind.
Don't snicker and don't stare.

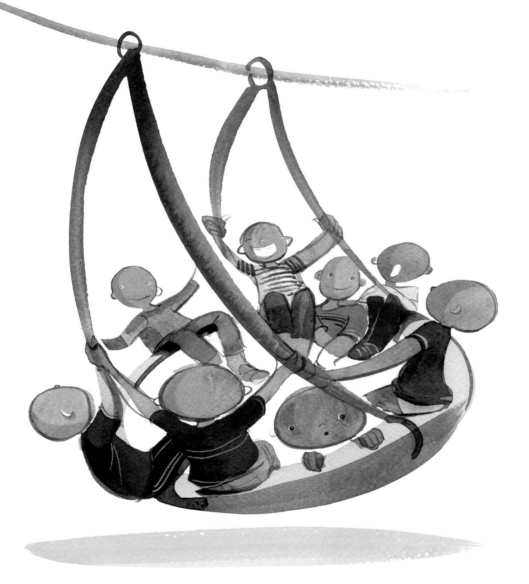

I'm thinking that's what you'd prefer
if your own head was bare.

It's hard to see her without hair.
I miss her curls that bounce.

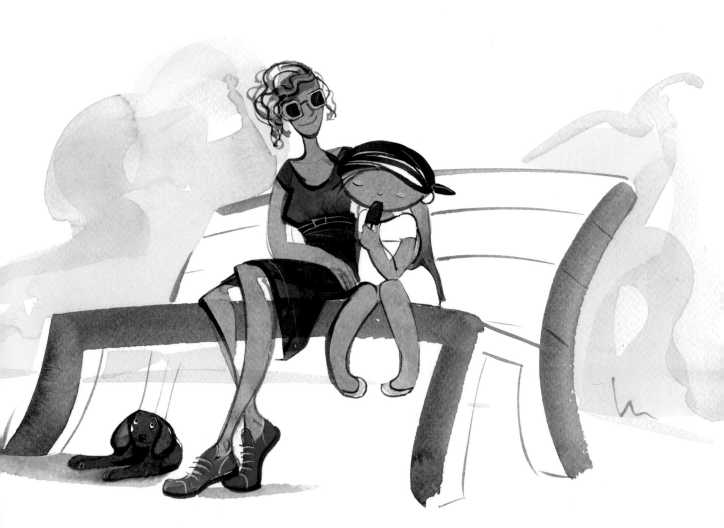

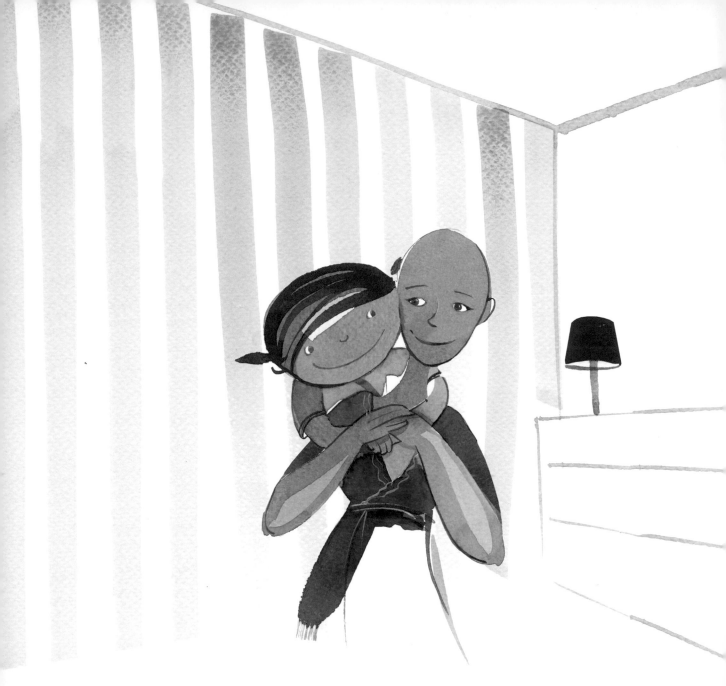

And though I know her hair will grow,
it's what's inside that counts.